This notebook belongs to

____

www.ingramcontent.com/pod-product-compliance
Lightning Source LLC
Chambersburg PA
CBHW072058280526
45788CB00006B/2322
9781092434232